JUST DATING.
NEWLYWEDS.
HAPPILY MARRIED.

EVERYONE WANTS
A NAUGHTY SEX LIFE...

SEX POSITIONS

SEX BUCKET LIST
for couples

100 SEXY POSITIONS AND NAUGHTY CHALLENGES

MADISON WEST

YOUR SEX LIFE WILL NEVER BE THE SAME!

the DIRTY CONTENTS

Rules Of The Game..7

The Sex Bucket List Pact 12

Chapter One: Virgin Territory................................... 13

Chapter Two: Heating Up...19

Chapter Three: Everything Oral............................... 34

Chapter Four: Sex, Sex, Sex...48

Chapter Five: Toys & Accesories................................87

Chapter Six: Playing In Public....................................95

Chapter Seven: Roleplay..100

Chapter Eight: Games...111

Bonus Chapter: At Your Own Risk.........................120

Top 5 Sex Challenges..125

Sexy Toy Wishlist..127

Your New Naughty Challenge................................129

REMEMBER, THIS IS CALLED A BUCKET LIST FOR A REASON.

THESE ARE THE THINGS YOU AND YOUR PARTNER SHOULD TRY AT LEAST ONCE IN YOUR LIFE!

AN OPEN MIND IS REQUIRED...

THE

Rules of the Game

EVERY GAME HAS RULES. THESE RULES ARE JUST A BIT MORE NAUGHTY.

RULE #1:

Welcome Back to Virginity

Or if you're actual virgins…
congrats- this book is going to be extra fun for you.

For all intents and purposes, every newlywed couple embarking on The Sex Bucket List must be pure, innocent virgins! Pretend (or embrace) that you are brand new to the sex game.

That means, you cannot go through the list crossing off dirty things that you've already done…because remember, you're officially virgins (again).

LOOPHOLE: If you'd like, you can go through this journal right now and cross out 10 things you've already done…

.a lot of. That way you can skip ahead to more thrilling adventures.

RULE 2:

Take Turns Choosing your Sexy Challenge

Just like foreplay, you don't have to go through this sex bucket list in any particular order. Let your sex drive do the picking. When a naughty opportunity presents itself or you get a certain urge to play out a fantasy – go for it.

RULE 3:

Push your Limits

Sexual enlightenment lies right outside of your erotic comfort zone. You're going to need an open mind and a willingness to be vulnerable.

Start slow and work your way up to the challenges that push you the most. Play by a "If you never try, you'll never know" mentality and just go with it.

If something feels weird, laugh about it together. Bond over it together. If something feels uncomfortable, tell your partner "Hey, this is new to me. Help me through this one". The whole point is to grow together and push your limits together.

LOOPHOLE #2: There may be a few things in this journal that are TOO outside of your sexual comfort zone. Together, feel free to cross something out if it doesn't fit into your relationship. Not sure about it? Leave it till the end. Who knows...you might be a freak by the end of this book.

RULE #4:

Keep Track. Keep Pace.

The best way to keep track of your Sex Bucket List is by using a highlighter to tick your adventures off before or after each escapade.

Make it a goal to tick off 3 challenges per week. By the end of the list, you'll have transformed your normal workweek into an exciting, passion-filled week with your partner.

In other words, don't take a year to complete this list! You'll lose all momentum.

THERE ARE 100 SEX BUCKET LIST CHALLENGES IN TOTAL...

To play, couples will wipe their sexual slate totally clean and start from the very beginning… welcome back to virginity.

You'll take turns choosing dirty positions and sexy fantasies to act out together. Discovering what turns each other on and exploring kinks you never knew you had. You'll be vulnerable. You'll be playful. And you'll create an intense bond with your partner on a much deeper level.

Plus, you've never cum this much in your life. I guarantee it….
It's time to break your sexual routine, discover what you've been missing, and put the play back into the bedroom.

You have full permission…no, I order you to get as dirty and freaky as you possibly can.

the

SEX BUCKET LIST

pact

Your first challenge starts now.

Grab each others' butts and say,

"LET'S HAVE SOME SEXY FUN".

Was that weird? Good.

Things are about to get a whole lot weirder.

Your first sexy experience starts now.

Remember, you don't have to go in order.
Let your libido do the picking…

CHAPTER ONE

VIRGIN TERRITORY

Do you remember the good ol' days of lingering foreplay?

The days when you were still holding onto your virginity and exploring your sexuality for hours at a time...over the clothes?

1 MAKE OUT - NO TOUCHING

Hands in neutral territory. Rediscover what it feels like to kiss your partner with no end goal in sight.

There's no rush to tear each other's clothes off or carry this situation to the bedroom.

the rule

After that kiss, walk away. And think about it for the rest of the day.

DONE!

RANKING:

Hers: 1   2   3   4   5   *His:*   1   2   3   4   5

WANNA DO IT AGAIN?   *Yes!!!*   *Nah...*

2 GRIND

Don't underestimate how hot and steamy this innocent little tease can be.

Get on top of your partner and start slowly kissing their neck and nibbling on their ear while you slowly begin to grind on their lap.

This will progress into a full-on make-out session.

the rule

No sex and nothing beneath the clothes. You've got to walk away like good little virgins.

DONE!

RANKING:

Hers: 1 2 3 4 5   *His:* 1 2 3 4 5

WANNA DO IT AGAIN?   *Yes!!!*   *Nah...*

3 SEXT!

Send each other dirty messages detailing everything. All-day long.

While you're both at work or school, send each other dirty messages detailing what you're going to do to each other once you get home.

the rule

Don't get upset if they don't respond right away, but they must respond before they come home from work or school.

DONE!

RANKING:

Hers: 1 2 3 4 5   *His:* 1 2 3 4 5

WANNA DO IT AGAIN? *Yes!!!*   *Nah...*

4 SEND A NAUGHTY PHOTO

Just a tease.
Leave a little to the imagination...
but not a lot.

the rule

Send this photo completely out of the blue. No warning.

DONE!

RANKING:

Hers: 1 2 3 4 5   *His:* 1 2 3 4 5

WANNA DO IT AGAIN?   *Yes!!!*   *Nah...*

5 NIBBLE EAR

You're either gonna love this or hate this.
Give it a shot.

the rule

Don't slobber like a dog.

DONE!

RANKING:

Hers: 1 2 3 4 5   *His:* 1 2 3 4 5

WANNA DO IT AGAIN?   *Yes!!!*   *Nah...*

CHAPTER TWO

HEATING UP

Things are gonna get a little bit weird
and a little bit naked.

6 SEXY OIL MASSAGE

Whoever snatches this challenge up first is lucky.

Not only do you get a full-body rub down with massage oils and lotions of your choosing, but you can also request a happy ending.

pro tip
Use intimate massage oil made to turn you on.

DONE!

RANKING:

Hers: 1 2 3 4 5   *His:* 1 2 3 4 5

WANNA DO IT AGAIN?   *Yes!!!*   *Nah...*

Ps. The best massage oil →

7 SEND A NAKED PIC

A dick pic. A titty pic.

Or whatever you love on your body, this is the time to show it off.

the rule

The recipient promises never to show this picture to anyone. Consider this legally binding.

DONE!

RANKING:

Hers: 1 2 3 4 5   *His:* 1 2 3 4 5

WANNA DO IT AGAIN? *Yes!!!*   *Nah...*

8   GIVE HIM A HANDJOB

Pro Tip: The key to a good hand job is lots of lube, whether that be KY lube, coconut oil, or spit.

Ask your man to show you how he likes it and where he likes to be touched OR tease him until he utterly cannot stand it anymore and is begging you to make him cum.

the rule

You cannot use your mouth to make him finish.

DONE!

RANKING:

Hers: 1 2 3 4 5   His: 1 2 3 4 5

WANNA DO IT AGAIN?   Yes!!!   Nah...

So much sexier with this...

9 MAKE HER CUM WITH JUST YOUR HANDS

A woman's vagina is like a combination lock; each one requires a different code to unlock. Learn that code!

Maybe she likes 2 fingers penetrating her or she might love you just rubbing her with your fingers.

the rule

Talk it out and don't be afraid!

DONE!

RANKING:

Hers: 1 2 3 4 5   His: 1 2 3 4 5

WANNA DO IT AGAIN? Yes!!!   Nah...

FUN FACT...

Sex can make you better when you're sick. Sexual arousal and orgasm are shown to boost your immune system and put your recuperation into turbo mode.

10 PHONE SEX

Anywhere, any time. Voice call your partner while they are at work and start talking dirty or call them while they're at a social function and tell them what you're doing to your body at that moment.

the rule

To be clear as to what is going on…don't be afraid to use the magic words, "Game on".

DONE!

RANKING:

Hers: 1 2 3 4 5   *His:* 1 2 3 4 5

WANNA DO IT AGAIN? *Yes!!!*   *Nah…*

11 VIDEO CALL

If you don't live together, this one will be easy. And if you do live together, go in separate rooms with each of your phones.

The person who picks this will call and instruct the other what he or she wants to see their partner do.

the rule

Clothes may be shed, toys may be used, and full-on orgasms may be had.

DONE!

RANKING:

Hers: 1 2 3 4 5   *His:* 1 2 3 4 5

WANNA DO IT AGAIN? *Yes!!!*   *Nah...*

12 PLAY WITH HER NIPPLES

Don't neglect this part of her body.
Use your tongue and your hand.
Ask her what she likes.

the rule

Take your time!

DONE!

RANKING:

Hers: 1 2 3 4 5   His: 1 2 3 4 5

WANNA DO IT AGAIN? *Yes!!!*   *Nah...*

SEXY FUN FACT...

Only around 25-30% of Women can orgasm from just penetration. That means almost 70% of women need clitoral stimulation to reach orgasm.

13 DESCRIBE IT

Now that you two have played with each other, it's time to communicate what you've enjoyed the most. And what you wanna do next.

The next time you're out at a restaurant, at a party, or even just across the table from one another, verbally describe – in detail- exactly what you want to do to your partner.

the rule

If you're having a hard time getting creative, make a "Top 3" list of dirty things you can't wait to act out.

DONE!

RANKING:

Hers: 1 2 3 4 5   *His:* 1 2 3 4 5

WANNA DO IT AGAIN? *Yes!!!*   *Nah...*

14 LET HER WATCH

His turn.
Give yourself a hand job while she watches.

the rule

She is not allowed to kiss you, to touch herself or to touch you. This is a one-man show.

DONE!

RANKING:

Hers: 1 2 3 4 5   *His:* 1 2 3 4 5

WANNA DO IT AGAIN? *Yes!!!*   *Nah...*

SEXY FUN FACT...

Hookups can lead to marriage…if you can get past that first night of weird sex. Actually, data shows that 1/3 of modern-day married couples started as a hookup.

15 LET HIM WATCH

Her turn. Lay back and please yourself just like you would alone. Do whatever it is that turns you on and let him study how you like to be touched and what brings you to orgasm.

the rule

The same rules apply. He is not allowed to kiss you, to touch himself, or to touch you. This is a one-man show.

DONE!

RANKING:

Hers: 1 2 3 4 5   *His:* 1 2 3 4 5

WANNA DO IT AGAIN? *Yes!!!*   *Nah...*

16 TAKE A BATH TOGETHER

Light some candles. Pour in some bubble bath. Put on some music. Dim the lights. Pop some bubbly. Really make this special. If something sexy doesn't happen in the bath, it certainly will once you dry off…

the rule

This is a good excuse to book a sexy hotel with a jacuzzi tub for the night.

DONE!

RANKING:

Hers: 1 2 3 4 5   *His:* 1 2 3 4 5

WANNA DO IT AGAIN? *Yes!!!*   *Nah…*

17 COOK NAKED

Ah, an easy one!

Whether one of you is baking cookies at home in the bare - and surprises the other. Or both of you decide to cook together without your clothes on...see how long you can last before dripping things on each other and licking them off.

the rule

An apron is allowed when around an open flame!

DONE!

RANKING:

Hers: 1 2 3 4 5   *His:* 1 2 3 4 5

WANNA DO IT AGAIN? *Yes!!!*   *Nah...*

18 FIND HIS G-SPOT

While you're giving your man a blow job, find his G-spot. Apply lube to your finger and very, very slowly insert your finger into his ass.

Move with his muscles as they allow you in; don't force it. About two inches in, move your finger upward in a "come hither" motion. Gently feel around to find his prostate which feels like a little jelly bean.

the rule

Don't force your fingers, just let it flow.

DONE!

RANKING:

Hers: 1 2 3 4 5   *His:* 1 2 3 4 5

WANNA DO IT AGAIN? *Yes!!!*   *Nah...*

SEXY FUN FACT...

Men have a G-spot, that super erogenous zone located right inside of his asshole. When stimulated by massaging or penetration, can provide euphoric sensations.

19 WATCH PORN TOGETHER

Take turns picking a porn. It doesn't matter the category.

Start out with the dramatic role-plays or PG stuff - these are the categories you can both giggle about together and get some new ideas. Go in the mindset that this is going to be an entertaining activity together...while we all know that it's impossible not to get turned on.

the rule

Eventually, start showing each other what you like to watch...and see how long you can go without turning the night into your own porno.

DONE!

RANKING:

Hers: 1 2 3 4 5   *His:* 1 2 3 4 5

WANNA DO IT AGAIN? *Yes!!!*   *Nah...*

CHAPTER THREE

EVERYTHING ORAL

Oral in bed is good, oral on the kitchen counter is even better.

Just by tweaking a few variables like the place and the position, you can create a brand new sexual experience for the both of you.

20 GO DOWN ON HER 'TIL SHE COMES

Eating a girl's pussy is like an Olympic sport. Each sport takes practice and dedication, just like a woman's gorgeous vagina. Making a woman cum with your tongue takes the right amount of pressure, speed, and time. Ask her what she likes.

Does she want you to go higher? Faster? Listen to the way she moans. Quiet might mean "change it up". Pay attention to how her body responds and you'll be able to give her a full-body orgasm that often comes with cunnilingus.

the rule

Most men don't know this, but sometimes a woman's inability to cum is that she's worried you're not enjoying it. So let her know you're not going to stop until she cums.

DONE!

RANKING:

Hers: 1 2 3 4 5   *His:* 1 2 3 4 5

WANNA DO IT AGAIN?   *Yes!!!*   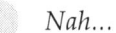   *Nah...*

21 GIVE HIM A BLOW-JOB

Orgasms from oral and orgasms from sex are 2 totally different experiences. Treat him to a relaxing and sensual BJ however you like it.

Play with that cock in new ways.
Lick it, spit on it, slap it against your tongue.

the rule

You can use your hands. In fact, I encourage you to.

DONE!

RANKING:

Hers: 1 2 3 4 5   *His:* 1 2 3 4 5

WANNA DO IT AGAIN? *Yes!!!*   *Nah...*

22 RIDE HIS FACE

There are two super sexy ways to ride your man's face.

ONE: Sit on his face and gently ride him. He'll love it.

TWO: Have him get on his knees while you put one leg up on the kitchen counter or desk. This will give him full access.

the rule

Girls, no pressure to come. Just get weird.

DONE!

RANKING:

Hers: 1   2   3   4   5   *His:*   1   2   3   4   5

WANNA DO IT AGAIN?   *Yes!!!*   *Nah...*

23 SIXTY-NINE

Him laying on his back, her straddling his face while his cock is perfectly positioned for her to play with - this mutual pleasure is the underrated sex position: 69.

the rule

Ladies, you can use your hands and your mouth here.

Guys, you can use your hands to move her back and forth on your face for some extra stimulation.

DONE!

RANKING:

Hers: 1 2 3 4 5   *His:* 1 2 3 4 5

WANNA DO IT AGAIN?   *Yes!!!*   *Nah...*

24 ORAL UNDER THE TABLE

While he's having his morning coffee at the table or she's in the middle of dinner, gracefully slide under the table and have fun.

the rule

Please do this in private. Duh!

DONE!

RANKING:

Hers: 1 2 3 4 5   *His:* 1 2 3 4 5

WANNA DO IT AGAIN?   *Yes!!!*   *Nah...*

SEXY FUN FACT...

Studies have shown that having sex with socks on increases the likelihood of an orgasm by 13-30%. Use non-slip socks for #SafetyFirst.

25 SWEET CUNNINGULUS

Chocolate Syrup, Ice Cream, Frosting – it's time for dessert. Here's the challenge: absolutely cover your girl's sweet spot in your sweet of choice. You're going to lick all of it up until they come.

the rule

Don't be afraid to make a mess. The best oral is always messy.

DONE!

RANKING:

Hers: 1 2 3 4 5   *His:* 1 2 3 4 5

WANNA DO IT AGAIN? *Yes!!!*   *Nah...*

Time to get messy...

26 THE LOLLIPOP BLOW-JOB

Ready to get messy?

Before you start sucking on him, start sucking on a lollipop while you get him started with your other hand. Watching you lick that sucker will get him instantly hard. After you've teased him enough, use all of that extra saliva and sticky juice in your mouth to give him the tastiest blow job ever – just don't put that lollipop down.

the rule

Stop once in a while to suck a little more, spit some of those juices all over his cock, and tease him while he begs for you to finish.

DONE!

RANKING:

Hers: 1 2 3 4 5   *His:* 1 2 3 4 5

WANNA DO IT AGAIN? *Yes!!!*   *Nah...*

The sexiest lollipops...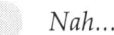

27 BLIND FOLDED BLOW-JOB

Use a tie or buy a satin mask for your girl to give you a blindfolded head.

Without her sight, she'll use all of her other senses to really get into it as she feels and tastes her way all over your cock.

the rule

She can take the blindfold off whenever she wants.

DONE!

RANKING:

Hers: 1 2 3 4 5 *His:* 1 2 3 4 5

WANNA DO IT AGAIN? *Yes!!!* *Nah...*

28 SWALLOW

For a man, having the tip of his cocked licked and sucked from the very beginning to the very end of a blow job is absolutely mind-blowing.

the rule

Let him finish in your mouth and it will be like the Christmas of oral sex.

DONE!

RANKING:

Hers: 1 2 3 4 5   His: 1 2 3 4 5

WANNA DO IT AGAIN? Yes!!!   Nah...

SEXY FUN FACT...

There are 36 calories in the average male ejaculation. Mmm protein.

29 BLOW-JOB... HE'S IN CONTROL

In this blow job, the man has all the power. You can make this as gentle or aggressive as you like- communicating as you go.

In this sexy play, the man grabs the woman by the back of her hair and guides her mouth up and down his cock just as he likes. For you naughty girls, have him push your head deep down onto his cock until it reaches the back of your throat. If you've never gagged on your man's dick, you're missing out.

the rule

She can say stop at any time.

DONE!

RANKING:

Hers: 1 2 3 4 5   *His:* 1 2 3 4 5

WANNA DO IT AGAIN? *Yes!!!*   *Nah...*

30 EAT HER ASS

It's the dawn of a new era in oral sex.
The asshole shall never be neglected again!

Girls, if you've never had your ass licked, holy hell you are in for a treat. And guys…we know that most of you have been wanting to do this for a while.

the rule

So, GAME ON!

DONE!

RANKING:

Hers: 1 2 3 4 5   *His:* 1 2 3 4 5

WANNA DO IT AGAIN? *Yes!!!*   *Nah…*

31/ GIVE HIM HEAD AND PLAY WITH YOURSELF

The Sex Bucket List mentions this a lot: the more pleasure you get-the more pleasure you give.

the rule

Girls, use a toy or use your fingers to have fun with yourself while you have fun with him.

DONE!

RANKING:

Hers: 1 2 3 4 5   His: 1 2 3 4 5

WANNA DO IT AGAIN? *Yes!!!*   *Nah...*

Ps. This is the best vibrator...

32 LUXURY BLOW-JOB

It's not just his cock that needs attention. The balls get neglected, mainly because us girls aren't taught what to do with them.

The man should be vocal in what he likes. Licking? Sucking? Cupping?

pro tip

To pay attention to his perineum — the nerve-packed area of skin between his balls and his butt. The girl can do this while he pleasures himself or takes a little break while giving him head.

DONE!

RANKING:

Hers: 1 2 3 4 5   *His:* 1 2 3 4 5

WANNA DO IT AGAIN? *Yes!!!*   *Nah...*

CHAPTER FOUR

SEX, SEX, SEX

Get ready for ALL of the positions in ALL of the places. Not only will these sexy ideas switch up your usual choreography of sexual positions, the adrenaline and sensation of new angles make each sexual experience feel like it's your first time.

33 SET THE MOOD

Get romantic with it.

Dim the lights, put on some 90's R&B, light some candles, and have sex…slowly. Do it right. Start with kissing. Touch gently.

the rule

Take your time to kiss every inch of each other's bodies.

DONE!

RANKING:

Hers: 1 2 3 4 5   *His:* 1 2 3 4 5

___

WANNA DO IT AGAIN? *Yes!!!*   *Nah…*

Candles that won't burn down your house. →

24 MORNING SEX

Wake your partner up with some slow touching and kissing- they'll get the hint.

pro tip

Morning sex is especially wonderful as a man's sex hormones are highest in the morning. Plus, why waste that morning wood?

DONE!

RANKING:

Hers: 1 2 3 4 5   *His:* 1 2 3 4 5

WANNA DO IT AGAIN? *Yes!!!*   *Nah...*

SEXY FUN FACT...

Simultaneous Orgasms are Rare. Pornos may have you believing that couples often cum at the same time, but this is actually extremely rare. Men come easier and more often than the woman. Make sure she's taken care of, too.

35 MIDDLE OF THE NIGHT SEX

The next time you stir in the night or get up to use the bathroom, use that moment as an opportunity to have blissful half-awake sex.

Your barely-coherent state makes for carnal sex where nothing is on your mind besides how badly your body wants it.

the rule

Don't forget to write in this journal in the morning.

DONE!

RANKING:

Hers: 1 2 3 4 5   *His:* 1 2 3 4 5

WANNA DO IT AGAIN? *Yes!!!*   *Nah...*

36 DOGGY STYLE

The angle of doggy is often one of the most pleasurable for both the man and the woman- hitting both of you in just the right spot.

Don't be afraid to add some variations in here: Ladies, you can have your man stay still as you back upon him with your own rhythm, giving you total control.

the rule

Try different speeds; fast and slow.

DONE!

RANKING:

Hers: 1 2 3 4 5   *His:* 1 2 3 4 5

WANNA DO IT AGAIN? *Yes!!!*   *Nah...*

37 INVOLVED DOGGY

Guys, slap that ass, pull her hair, and rub on her asshole with some spit.

You've got access to lots of stimulating activities back there.

the rule

Listen to what she likes.

DONE!

RANKING:

Hers: 1 2 3 4 5   *His:* 1 2 3 4 5

WANNA DO IT AGAIN? *Yes!!!*   *Nah...*

38 PILLOW ASSIST

Missionary with some height.

Put a pillow under her hips to get even deeper.

the rule

You can push her legs back even further for total control.

DONE!

RANKING:

Hers: 1 2 3 4 5   *His:* 1 2 3 4 5

WANNA DO IT AGAIN? *Yes!!!*   *Nah...*

The best sex accessory you never knew you needed...

39. MISSIONARY & CLITORAL STIMULATION

This one sounds like the title of a Broadway play… and trust me, it will be just as dramatic.

While the man slowly penetrates the woman, she'll rub her clit with her eyes closed, just like she masturbates solo. As she gets close to orgasm, her juices will drench his cock.

pro tip

When the moment finally approaches, he will feel her contracting all around him as he gets close to finishing as well.

DONE!

RANKING:

Hers: 1 2 3 4 5   *His:* 1 2 3 4 5

WANNA DO IT AGAIN?   *Yes!!!*   *Nah…*

40 SEX AFTER SHE COMES

Whether she cums from oral, clitoral stimulation, masturbation, or straight-up penetration- the sensation of being fucked while still cumming can oftentimes provide a woman with either an elongated orgasm or multiple orgasms.

the rule

Just be wary of her clit; it might be sensitive.

DONE!

RANKING:

Hers: 1 2 3 4 5   *His:* 1 2 3 4 5

WANNA DO IT AGAIN? *Yes!!!*   *Nah...*

41 COWGIRL

Ladies on top.

Hold on to the headboard or put your hands on his chest as you ride him.

pro tip

This position is fantastic for hitting your g-spot.

DONE!

RANKING:

Hers: 1 2 3 4 5   *His:* 1 2 3 4 5

WANNA DO IT AGAIN? *Yes!!!*   *Nah...*

43 FROGGY

I know, I know...this doesn't sound very sexy, but he's going to love it. You can try a froggy variation to give you even more control as you put your feet flat on the mattress or floor. Now you can do mini squats up and down on his hard cock.

pro tip

This position is fantastic for hitting your g-spot.

DONE!

RANKING:

Hers: 1 2 3 4 5   His: 1 2 3 4 5

WANNA DO IT AGAIN? *Yes!!!*   *Nah...*

44 STILL COWGIRL

Just like it sounds, she's on top but doesn't move.

Instead, he holds her hips and thrusts in and out and she enjoys the ride.

the rule

Only he can move.

DONE!

RANKING:

Hers: 1 2 3 4 5   His: 1 2 3 4 5

WANNA DO IT AGAIN? *Yes!!!*   *Nah...*

45 REVERSE COWGIRL

This one takes some practice (and some balance).

Reverse cowgirl is when the woman is on top, but facing away from the man. Sometimes this position can be tricky for the woman to move her hips up and down- so instead, let the man try pumping up into her.

the rule

Use your hands to balance; hold on to his legs or put your hands flat on the mattress between his legs.

DONE!

RANKING:

Hers: 1 2 3 4 5   *His:* 1 2 3 4 5

WANNA DO IT AGAIN? *Yes!!!*   *Nah...*

46 USE LOTS OF LUBE

Sex with proper lube is like an other-worldly experience. Everything is more sensitive and you're able to try a lot of tight positions that may not have worked before. Many studies have shown that using lube can help increase the likelihood of having an orgasm by 50%. Those odds are just too good not to try.

the rule

You can try KY lube or coconut oil which are both long-lasting forms of lube, rather than just using spit or relying on natural body lubrication.

DONE!

RANKING:

Hers: 1 2 3 4 5   His: 1 2 3 4 5

WANNA DO IT AGAIN? *Yes!!!*   *Nah...*

Get ready for a new level of sex with this....

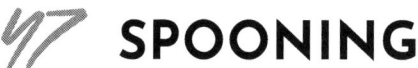 SPOONING

This is one of those positions where lube makes a world of difference! Get into the spooning position.

The man will slide his hard cock between her legs for the perfect angle of penetration. He can hold her waist or legs for extra leverage.

the rule

She can wrap one leg over his legs for extra deep access.

DONE!

RANKING:

Hers: 1 2 3 4 5   *His:* 1 2 3 4 5

WANNA DO IT AGAIN? *Yes!!!*   *Nah...*

48 LET HIM CUM WHEREVER HE WANTS

Tits, ass, stomach, face… get creative.

Just when he is about to cum, he'll let you know as he gets in position to hit his target.

the rule

Don't get it in her hair.

DONE!

RANKING:

Hers: 1 2 3 4 5 His: 1 2 3 4 5

WANNA DO IT AGAIN? Yes!!! Nah…

49 CHOKE HER

Not too hard and not too soft and not for too long. Start out with 5 seconds at a time.

This is just the right amount of time to restrict a bit of oxygen to the brain, giving the woman a euphoric sensation all over her body.

the rule

You're lightly targeting her airway, not her vocal box.

DONE!

RANKING:

Hers: 1 2 3 4 5   *His:* 1 2 3 4 5

WANNA DO IT AGAIN?   *Yes!!!*   *Nah...*

50 SPANKING

Spankings go both ways. Whoever chooses this Sex Bucket List item decides who gets the spankings.

Maybe you want them lightly or maybe you want your ass to be full of red handprints. Find that balance together.

the rule

You can use your hand, a paddle, a belt, a wooden spoon... get creative, and don't be afraid to check out some toys on Amazon.

DONE!

RANKING:

Hers: 1 2 3 4 5   *His:* 1 2 3 4 5

WANNA DO IT AGAIN? *Yes!!!*   *Nah...*

51 PULL HER HAIR

There is a proper and improper way to pull a woman's hair.

IMPROPER: Grabbing her hair by the ends or the end of her ponytail and yanking on it, causing her neck to experience whiplash.

PROPER: Grabbing a handful of hair by the root and holding your hand in place- the pulling comes along naturally as your bodies move together.

the rule

Pull her hair during sex, during blowjobs, or to initiate a dominant move will bring out her submissive side.

DONE!

RANKING:

Hers: 1 2 3 4 5   His: 1 2 3 4 5

WANNA DO IT AGAIN? *Yes!!!*   *Nah...*

52 ROUGH SEX

Once you two have established how much hair-pulling you like, how much choking you can handle, and how hard to slap each other's asses: go for it.

the rule

Pin him up against the wall, throw her on the bed...and if you like, add a little light slapping and dirty talk in the mix.

DONE!

RANKING:

Hers: ① ② ③ ④ ⑤   *His:* ① ② ③ ④ ⑤

WANNA DO IT AGAIN? *Yes!!!*   *Nah...*

The rough sex starter kit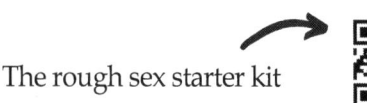

53 SEX ON THE STAIRS

The angles you can get on the stairs are magical! Doggy, cowgirl, acrobatic bending and twisting.

the rule

Just be sure to get busy at the bottom of the stairs….!

DONE!

RANKING:

Hers: 1 2 3 4 5   *His:* 1 2 3 4 5

WANNA DO IT AGAIN?   *Yes!!!*   *Nah…*

54 SEX ON THE FLOOR

While a mattress has a bit of bounce that moves with you, the floor gives you total control during sex and allows you to get a bit deeper.

pro tip

The floor is particularly fantastic for any kind of cowgirl position!

DONE!

RANKING:

Hers: 1 2 3 4 5   His: 1 2 3 4 5

WANNA DO IT AGAIN?   Yes!!!   Nah...

SEXY FUN FACT...

According to Porn Hub data, Utah is the kinkiest state in terms of the taboo stuff that residents like to watch. But that's not really hard to believe, is it?

55 LEGS UP

To get the deepest possible penetration, the woman will lay in her back and put her ankles on her man's shoulders.

the rule

Start slow. Super slow.

DONE!

RANKING:

Hers: 1 2 3 4 5   *His:* 1 2 3 4 5

WANNA DO IT AGAIN? *Yes!!!*   *Nah...*

56 LEGS UP: VERSION 2

This is an even more intense variation to Legs Up. The man grabs both her ankles and puts them on one shoulder.

Grabbing both legs helps him pull her even deeper towards him.

the rule

Again...start slow. This gets really deep.

DONE!

RANKING:

Hers: 1 2 3 4 5   *His:* 1 2 3 4 5

WANNA DO IT AGAIN? *Yes!!!*   *Nah...*

57 GIRLS, ONE KNEE UP

Lay in missionary. Girls, pull one knee to your chest for deeper pleasure.

the rule

This angle allows you to play with yourself more easily.

DONE!

RANKING:

Hers: 1 2 3 4 5   *His:* 1 2 3 4 5

WANNA DO IT AGAIN? *Yes!!!*   *Nah...*

58 AGAINST THE WALL

Girls, bend over. Hands on the wall.
Your man will be behind you in a new form of doggy.

the rule

Watch your face.

DONE!

RANKING:

Hers: 1 2 3 4 5   *His:* 1 2 3 4 5

WANNA DO IT AGAIN? *Yes!!!*   *Nah...*

59 SEX IN THE SHOWER

Start by soaping each other up – a loofa is a worthy investment for this sexy play spot. Rub soap all over her beautiful breasts and pour bath gel all down his chest.

the rule

When it comes time for full-on sex, try a version of doggy where she uses the wall as support or the man can sit on the shower floor while she rides him using his shoulders for leverage.

DONE!

RANKING:

Hers: 1 2 3 4 5   *His:* 1 2 3 4 5

WANNA DO IT AGAIN? *Yes!!!*   *Nah...*

Get extra soapy...

60 LAZY SEX

Ladies, lay on your stomach, legs closed. Your man will slide in between your thighs to penetrate you with extra friction.

the rule

Don't forget the lube.

DONE!

RANKING:

Hers: 1 2 3 4 5   *His:* 1 2 3 4 5

WANNA DO IT AGAIN?   *Yes!!!*   *Nah...*

SEXY FUN FACT...

Sex is good for you! When you have sex, especially with your partner, your body releases endorphins, adrenaline, serotonin, and promotes healthy circulation. These benefits lead to less stress, healthier hearts, and decrease depression.

61 NETFLIX & CHILL

This is a marathon of sex while you watch a marathon of your favorite show. Stay in bed all day, or all night.

the rule

At least 3 sexual activities must be completed.

DONE!

RANKING:

Hers: 1 2 3 4 5   *His:* 1 2 3 4 5

WANNA DO IT AGAIN?   *Yes!!!*   *Nah...*

62 SEX IN THE KITCHEN

Bend her over the kitchen table first and then throw her on top of the counter.

The cool surfaces on her tits and ass will bring new sensations to her body while the different level positions provide fabulous angles for penetration.

the rule

Test the sturdiness of surfaces before you fuck on them

DONE!

RANKING:

Hers: 1 2 3 4 5   *His:* 1 2 3 4 5

WANNA DO IT AGAIN?   *Yes!!!*   *Nah...*

63. SEX ON A CHAIR

Have the man sit ass-naked on a chair.

This can be a kitchen table chair with no arms or a big lazy boy-style chair.

the rule

Test the chair's strength before you start.

DONE!

RANKING:

Hers: 1 2 3 4 5   *His:* 1 2 3 4 5

WANNA DO IT AGAIN? *Yes!!!*   *Nah...*

64 A QUICKIE

Mastering the art of quickies is key to a healthy sex life.

Get those endorphins pumping and those serotonin levels flowing with a quick 5-10 minute bang.

the rule

Take pleasure in knowing that the two of you desire each other so badly that you'll take every morsel you can get.

DONE!

RANKING:

Hers: 1 2 3 4 5   *His:* 1 2 3 4 5

WANNA DO IT AGAIN? *Yes!!!* *Nah...*

65 ANAL

Anal is something that takes a lot of care and practice.

Many girls who LOVE anal report that it took them 2-3 times to enjoy it, but they were committed to the cause because mentally, they liked the idea.

the rule

Start out with your fingers and lots of lube. When your ass is ready, have your man slowly put in just the tip. Relax. Go slow. Very slow. Don't be a hero.

DONE!

RANKING:

Hers: 1 2 3 4 5   *His:* 1 2 3 4 5

WANNA DO IT AGAIN? *Yes!!!*   *Nah...*

First practice playing with these... →

66 SEX IN FRONT OF A MIRROR

Bent over the bathroom sink in front of the mirror, on the floor in front of the closet mirror, or moving a mirror next to the bed for the perfect view…watching yourself fuck and be fucked is next-level good.

the rule

Just be aware, it's totally normal not to like every angle! Just like you're taking a photo, position yourself in a way that makes you feel sexy.

DONE!

RANKING:

Hers: 1 2 3 4 5   His: 1 2 3 4 5

WANNA DO IT AGAIN? Yes!!!   Nah…

67 TALK DIRTY

Dirty talk comes naturally to some and is really difficult for others.

So, here's how I want you to think of this: you're basically narrating your sex. Ask each other questions like, "Do you like when I [insert current action here]" or "Yes, I love it when you [insert motion here]" or even tell your partner what you're about to do like, "I'm going to [insert sex act here] now".

the rule

Laugh, it's okay!

DONE!

RANKING:

Hers: 1 2 3 4 5   *His:* 1 2 3 4 5

WANNA DO IT AGAIN?   *Yes!!!*   *Nah...*

68 HANDS BEHIND HER BACK

In any position, the girl will put her hands behind her back. Her man will grab her wrists for control while he fucks her.

the rule

Make sure not to hurt her...unless she wants you to.

DONE!

RANKING:

Hers: 1 2 3 4 5   *His:* 1 2 3 4 5

WANNA DO IT AGAIN? *Yes!!!*   *Nah...*

69 SHE'S IN CONTROL

Men, you are to be totally submissive as your woman directs you in every position she desires.

the rule

Guys, let go of control.

DONE!

RANKING:

Hers: 1 2 3 4 5   *His:* 1 2 3 4 5

WANNA DO IT AGAIN? *Yes!!!*   *Nah...*

70 PUNISH

Whether she's been a bad girl, or he's been a bad boy, it's time for some punishment. This one involves dirty talk and spankings.

the rule

Know your limits.

DONE!

RANKING:

Hers: 1 2 3 4 5   *His:* 1 2 3 4 5

WANNA DO IT AGAIN? *Yes!!!*   *Nah...*

71 FINGERS IN HER MOUTH

In missionary or in doggy, put your fingers in her mouth while you fuck her.

the rule

Make sure your finger are kinda clean...

DONE!

RANKING:

Hers: 1 2 3 4 5   *His:* 1 2 3 4 5

WANNA DO IT AGAIN? *Yes!!!*   *Nah...*

CHAPTER FIVE

TOYS & ACCESORIES

There is a reason that sex toys are so popular: because they make sex feel awesome. Vibrating sensations, a little bit of pain, more orgasms, and free hands that were previously occupied. It's time to see what all of the fuss is about...

72 TEASE HER WITH A VIBRATOR

Game. Changer. Curved vibrators can stimulate her g-spot, can be used to tease her nipples, and are magic at getting her to a clitoral orgasm. The vibrator can be used by her partner as he explores what makes her body shake or it can be used by her to have a full orgasm while her man is penetrating her during sex.

Having a vibrator in the mix can easily double the amount of orgasms a girl has during sex with her partner. Over and over again.

the rule

Play with the vibrator until she comes.

DONE!

RANKING:

Hers: 1 2 3 4 5   *His:* 1 2 3 4 5

WANNA DO IT AGAIN? *Yes!!!* *Nah...*

73. VIBRATOR FOR HER DURING SEX

While you fuck her, she's going to use a vibrator on herself.

the rule

She cums first.

DONE!

RANKING:

Hers: 1 2 3 4 5   *His:* 1 2 3 4 5

WANNA DO IT AGAIN? *Yes!!!*   *Nah...*

A smaller, handheld vibrator like this is easier to incorpate while the two of you are having sex.

74 GIRLS, DRESS UP

Girls, it's time to get extra slutty.

Buy some fishnet stockings, a sexy bra, and put on some red lipstick.

the rule

Prepare for those fish nets to be ripped and that lipstick to be smeared.

DONE!

RANKING:

Hers: 1 2 3 4 5   *His:* 1 2 3 4 5

WANNA DO IT AGAIN? *Yes!!!*   *Nah...*

75 GUYS, DRESS UP

Guys, you can be silly with a YMCA outfit or you get serious with a suit and tie. Your choice.

the rule

Make it a surprise.

DONE!

RANKING:

Hers: ① ② ③ ④ ⑤ *His:* ① ② ③ ④ ⑤

WANNA DO IT AGAIN? *Yes!!!*   *Nah...*

SEXY FUN FACT...

Sex is better in a relationship. One night stands don't give you the opportunity to learn about the other persons preferences; you kind of just flop around. Studies have shown that love makes the difference between mediocre sex and mind-blowing sex.

76 A LEATHER PADDLE FOR SPANKING

Finding the line between pleasure and pain is an acquired skill. Find that balance, and your body releases opiate-like endorphins that give you a sexual high. Spanking is the perfect activity to cause this reaction.

When you're spanking, you want to hit the juiciest part of the cheeks – usually right at the crease of the ass and leg. Spank in slightly different spots to cause more of a slapping sensation.

the rule

Keep hitting the same spot to create more pain. The anticipation between each spanking is so arousing for the one being punished.

DONE!

RANKING:

Hers: 1 2 3 4 5   *His:* 1 2 3 4 5

WANNA DO IT AGAIN?   *Yes!!!*   *Nah...*

Ps. Use this...

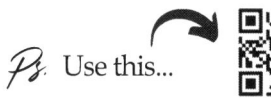

77 HANDCUFFS

Whether you're incorporating cold metal handcuffs into a cops & robber situation or you surprise your partner with fuzzy or silicone handcuffs that restrain their hands behind their back while you tease them relentlessly.

pro tip

...handcuffs are a quick and easy way to turn regular Wednesday-night sex into a world of fantasy.

DONE!

RANKING:

Hers: 1 2 3 4 5   *His:* 1 2 3 4 5

WANNA DO IT AGAIN? *Yes!!!*   *Nah...*

You're welcome. →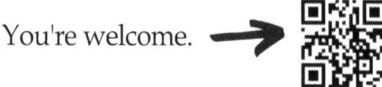

78 TIES FOR THE BED POSTS

The submissive partner in this scenario will be totally vulnerable to his or her partner, which heightens the sensation of every touch, every kiss, and every instance of penetration.

Add a blindfold in the mix for an even more intense sexual experience. The dominant partner has total control, having his or her way with a helplessly restrained sex toy.

the rule

He or she can let their carnal desires dictate how rough or sensual they will play.

DONE!

RANKING:

Hers: 1 2 3 4 5   *His:* 1 2 3 4 5

WANNA DO IT AGAIN?   *Yes!!!*   *Nah...*

These won't break your headboard.

CHAPTER SIX

PLAYING IN PUBLIC

That feeling of doing something dirty at the risk of getting caught can be such a turn on. The delayed gratification of slow foreplay and the buildup to hot and heavy sex is something that every couple should experience together.

79 SEXT AT DINNER

Go to a nice restaurant. One where you should be on your best, if not decent, behavior. Start with a couple of dirty texts at the table. Text each other what you want to do at that moment and watch your partner squirm with excitement.

At some point in the night, both of you will take a turn going to the bathroom and sending a naughty photo to the other, which must be opened discreetly at the table.

the rule

Fuck each other with your eyes and then when you get back to the car, take a few minutes to release some of that sexual tension.

DONE!

RANKING:

Hers: 1 2 3 4 5   His: 1 2 3 4 5

WANNA DO IT AGAIN? Yes!!!   Nah...

80 REMOTE CONTROL VIBRATOR

At dinner, he can increase the vibrator's speed and change up the settings whenever and wherever he likes to watch her squirm.

pro tip

The vibrator is small enough that she may even forget that it's inside of her...at least until you turn it on.

DONE!

RANKING:

Hers: 1 2 3 4 5   *His:* 1 2 3 4 5

WANNA DO IT AGAIN? *Yes!!!*   *Nah...*

 ← In...or out. →

81 FINGER HER IN THE CAR

To get ready for this naughty play, wear a skirt or a dress; something with easy access.

Start by rubbing and then slide a few fingers in when she's really wet.

pro tip

If you don't have tinted windows, you'll have to be sneaky about this one.

DONE!

RANKING:

Hers: 1 2 3 4 5   *His:* 1 2 3 4 5

WANNA DO IT AGAIN? *Yes!!!*   *Nah...*

82 BLOW JOB IN THE CAR

Pull over on a secluded road. Emphasis on secluded!

We're talking back-roads in the forest! The man stays where he is while the lady leans over to play.

adult warning

I really don't want you to get in trouble with this one so make sure you're at no risk of being caught.

DONE!

RANKING:

Hers: 1 2 3 4 5   *His:* 1 2 3 4 5

WANNA DO IT AGAIN? *Yes!!!*   *Nah...*

CHAPTER SEVEN

ROLE PLAY

We all have a fantasy, but some of us are too shy to ask for it.

That's why I am here to MAKE YOU step into fantasy land.

83 CAMPING SEX

Pitch a literal tent in the backyard or in the wilderness for a night of wild sex.

The change of scenery is thrilling and the lack of distractions is extremely intimate. Whether you're having loud passionate sex with the acoustics of the forest or having to muffle her screams so that your camping neighbors don't hear, camping sex is hot. Remember... this is your real-life porno.

pro tip

Bring towels and baby wipes to clean up the mess as you might not have access to a shower.

DONE!

RANKING:

Hers: 1 2 3 4 5   *His:* 1 2 3 4 5

WANNA DO IT AGAIN? *Yes!!!* *Nah...*

84 LET HER CALL YOU DADDY

Let me explain this one: you're not her actual daddy!

But you are the man who controls her, who tells her she's "a good girl" or "a bad girl". You're the man who rewards her with kisses or punishes her with spankings.

the rule

Try the words, "yes, daddy" and "no, daddy" – and see where that takes you.

DONE!

RANKING:

Hers: 1 2 3 4 5   *His:* 1 2 3 4 5

WANNA DO IT AGAIN? *Yes!!!*   *Nah...*

85 THE REPAIR MAN

Have a leaky shower?

Better call the repairman over to use his big tools to fix it.

pro tip

Make sure to test out the shower yourself before he leaves. Oh no...you can't find your wallet? How ever are you going to pay him?

DONE!

RANKING:

Hers: 1 2 3 4 5   *His:* 1 2 3 4 5

WANNA DO IT AGAIN? *Yes!!!*   *Nah...*

86 STRANGERS IN A BAR

Pick a bar that you've never been to before.

Dress in a sexy outfit that you don't usually wear. Sit separately and then ask the bartender to send the cute girl or sexy man at the other end of the bar a shot. So surprised by this gesture, you'll certainly get an invite to join.

the rule

Spark up a conversation about where you're from and what you're doing at such a lonely bar on your own. Perhaps, you two can keep each other company for the rest of the night...

DONE!

RANKING:

Hers: 1 2 3 4 5 *His:* 1 2 3 4 5

WANNA DO IT AGAIN? *Yes!!!* *Nah...*

87 CLIENT AND CALL GIRL...OR CALL BOY

Let your call girl know that you'd like to reserve her services for a couple of hours.

Text her the address of the hotel and your room number. Tell her what you want her to wear and what you are planning to do to her (or what you want her to do to you) once she arrives.

the rule

When she knocks on the door of your hotel room, the ultimate fantasy begins. She is there to cater to your every need and desire.

DONE!

RANKING:

Hers: 1 2 3 4 5   *His:* 1 2 3 4 5

WANNA DO IT AGAIN? *Yes!!!*   *Nah...*

88 UBER DRIVER

You'll need a ride home after your night out with the guys or maybe when you've locked your keys in your car at work.

Text your "Uber Driver" and a car will be there shortly. Get in the back seat. Once you notice how attractive your driver is, you might start to feel turned on and even need to start touching yourself during the ride. Ask your driver to take a detour to a secluded area and ask them to join you in the back seat.

pro tip

Or maybe once you get to your destination, get into the front seat and pull your driver towards you to initiate some steamy car sex.

DONE!

RANKING:

Hers: 1 2 3 4 5   *His:* 1 2 3 4 5

WANNA DO IT AGAIN? *Yes!!!*   *Nah...*

89 MASTER & SLAVE

Whips, belts, ties, and brazen commands…the slave must concede to every one of the Master's wishes. The slave is utterly submissive and obeys every single word.

Of course, pick out a safe word. The "safe word" doesn't always mean stop, it can also be a signal just to slow it down or ease up a little.

the rule

Keep a steady pace of pain with communication.

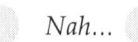

RANKING:

Hers: 1 2 3 4 5   *His:* 1 2 3 4 5

WANNA DO IT AGAIN? *Yes!!!*   *Nah…*

90 THE SEXY MAID

Bending over in that short maid's skirt to dust the lamp with a feather duster. On your hands and knees to wipe the floors.

Spilling water all over your chest while doing the dishes. Being a maid can be a messy and physical job.

the rule

If she isn't cleaning to the homeowner's satisfaction, there may be some punishment involved.

DONE!

RANKING:

Hers: 1 2 3 4 5   *His:* 1 2 3 4 5

WANNA DO IT AGAIN? *Yes!!!*   *Nah...*

Just an idea...

91 PORN STARS

Pick a porn that you really love …we all have one.

And reenact it scene by scene.
Don't skip any position, ass slap, or deep kiss.

the rule

Really get into the role.

DONE!

RANKING:

Hers: 1 2 3 4 5   *His:* 1 2 3 4 5

WANNA DO IT AGAIN? *Yes!!!*   *Nah…*

92 DOCTOR & PATIENT

Not feeling well? Don't worry, your doctor is here to examine your entire body, head to toe, to diagnose the issue, and treat you with some TLC.

Stay in character by choosing a name for the patient, like Mr. Clark, and stick to calling the other partner 'Doctor'.

the rule

Use these words as often as you can to really put yourselves into the scene.

DONE!

RANKING:

Hers: 1 2 3 4 5   His: 1 2 3 4 5

WANNA DO IT AGAIN? *Yes!!!*   *Nah...*

CHAPTER EIGHT

GAMES

Sex doesn't always have to be serious. Sex can be fun, too. In fact, laughter and a sense of play help break the tension during new sexual experiences. Playing games and goofing around will bring you both out of your shell, allowing you to try new things and push each others' erotic boundaries comfortably.

93 SILENT SEX

Sounds easy, right? Wrong. Try fucking without making a sound. Do what you have to do, bite your lip, cover her mouth, shove her face into a pillow… all are fair game.

To ramp up the stakes, whenever one of you makes a noise – the other person has to totally stop what they're doing.

the rule

You'll discover that when you're not allowed to expresses yourself verbally or vocally, you find another way to let that pleasure out through biting, squeezing, and desperately grabbing your partner.

DONE!

RANKING:

Hers: 1 2 3 4 5   *His:* 1 2 3 4 5

WANNA DO IT AGAIN? *Yes!!!*   *Nah…*

94 THIRTY SECONDS

Set a timer for 30 seconds. In this time, the Woman will take her turn having her way with her Man.

She can do whatever she wants to his body for 30 seconds. When the timer goes off, switch. Set a goal for how long you want to play this game.

the rule

Take turns each for a few minutes. By the end, you'll be dying to take each other.

DONE!

RANKING:

Hers: 1 2 3 4 5 *His:* 1 2 3 4 5

WANNA DO IT AGAIN? *Yes!!!*   *Nah...*

95 HIDE & GO FUCK

The adult version of Hide and Go Seek: One person goes and hides somewhere in the house or the yard while the other person counts to 30.

The hider better pick a good spot...because when the seeker finds them - the seeker fucks them.

the rule

Everyone has to be naked.

DONE!

RANKING:

Hers: 1 2 3 4 5   *His:* 1 2 3 4 5

WANNA DO IT AGAIN? *Yes!!!*   *Nah...*

96 NAUGHTY TRUTH-OR-DARE

We all know how this game goes. Feel free to search the web for some ideas beforehand. Here are some Truths and Dares to get you started…

TRUTH:
"What have you always wanted to try sexually?"
"What's your favorite thing that I do to your body?"

DARE:
"I dare you to give me a sexy strip tease to any song of my choice".
"I dare you to take my underwear off with your teeth"

the rule

No changing your choice of Truth or Dare!

DONE!

RANKING:

Hers: 1 2 3 4 5   His: 1 2 3 4 5

WANNA DO IT AGAIN? *Yes!!!*   *Nah...*

97 SEX DICE

When you can add laughter and playfulness into the bedroom, it takes the pressure off of sex or being sexy! Grab a glass of wine and roll with it.

the rule

You must obey the dice.

DONE!

RANKING:

Hers: 1 2 3 4 5   *His:* 1 2 3 4 5

WANNA DO IT AGAIN? *Yes!!!*   *Nah...*

Get Them Here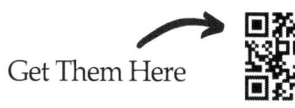

98 STRIP POKER

Or Strip Chess. Or Strip Checkers. Or Strip BattleShip. You can turn any game into a stripping game if you just believe in yourself.

This kind of playful spirit brings out the flirt in both of you. The tease of watching clothes slowly coming off is wonderfully torturous. And that competitive edge will add a little spice to your dynamic.

the rule

If you want to step the game up one more level, you can make a rule that whoever is naked first receives a penalty of some slutty sex act or spankings.

DONE!

RANKING:

Hers: 1 2 3 4 5   *His:* 1 2 3 4 5

WANNA DO IT AGAIN? *Yes!!!*   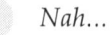   *Nah...*

99 SEXY ART

Ready to get messy and creative? Buy a white canvas (or something you can paint on) and some paint. Get naked, paint each other up and create your own sexy art piece.

Hang it on your wall. It will be your little secret to keep when people comment on how much they love your Avant Gard art.

pro tip

Lay down a tarp first!

DONE!

RANKING:

Hers: 1 2 3 4 5   His: 1 2 3 4 5

WANNA DO IT AGAIN? Yes!!!   Nah...

100 TARZAN & JANE

Bringing the animal kingdom to the bedroom, things are about to get rough in this male pursuit/female resistance game.

Secure ropes or ties to the corners of the bed. The goal is for Tarzan to wrestle Jane into submission, getting both of her hands and legs tightly secured. Jane's job is to resist.

pro tip

While this 'Tarzan and Jane' might sound rapey, with a partner that you trust, this game can be so hot. It starts out playful and funny, then all of a sudden, your inner animal is unleashed and you end up having super hot rough sex.

DONE!

RANKING:

Hers: 1 2 3 4 5   His: 1 2 3 4 5

WANNA DO IT AGAIN? *Yes!!!*   *Nah...*

BONUS CHAPTER

AT YOUR OWN RISK

Everything in this chapter has gotten me negative reviews for being "too hardcore".

My bad.

If you're sex life is fulfilled, stop reading now. But if you wanna get super freaky, keep reding.

101 RIM JOB

For a man. the idea of asking for a girl to lick his ass feels so taboo.

So he may never ask.
But I'm asking you to try it.

the rule

Take an intermission during a blow-job to do this.

DONE!

RANKING:

Hers: 1 2 3 4 5   His: 1 2 3 4 5

WANNA DO IT AGAIN? *Yes!!!*   *Nah...*

102 VISIT A STRIP CLUB

Instead of going to a bar or a club…you're going to a titty bar.

Get a little boozy or stay stone cold sober and watch some naked girls together. When you get back to the car, you'll be dying to touch each other.

the rule

Set boundaries before you go: are lap dances allowed?

DONE!

RANKING:

Hers: 1 2 3 4 5   *His:* 1 2 3 4 5

WANNA DO IT AGAIN?   *Yes!!!*   *Nah…*

103 VISIT A SWINGERS CLUB

Every big city has one.

A club where couples or solo kinks visit to either watch other people have sex or to join in on some group fun.

the rule

If you two are really kinky, you can plan on finding another couple to swap with. Alternatively, you can plan to just go there and watch; your preference will be respected here.
OR you can go with no plan and see what happens.

DONE!

RANKING:

Hers: 1 2 3 4 5   *His:* 1 2 3 4 5

WANNA DO IT AGAIN?   *Yes!!!*   *Nah...*

104 HAVE A THREESOME

This is called a Bucket List for a reason! These are the crazy sexual experiences that you should have at least once before you die!

For your first threesome, it's easier to involve a stranger.

Get on Tinder and set up a couple's profile. Or go out to a bar with the idea of picking up a 3rd party.

the rule

Set some boundaries first. Is he allowed to kiss the 3rd party on the mouth? Are the 2 of you going to share the 3rd party? Or is the 3rd party going to share the woman? Watch some threesome pornos to see what you like.

DONE!

RANKING:

Hers: 1 2 3 4 5   *His:* 1 2 3 4 5

WANNA DO IT AGAIN? *Yes!!!*   *Nah...*

FINISHED
THE CHALLENGE?

You dirty kids.

But hey, you're not done yet.

Now both of you need to scan through the past 100 sexual experiences and pick your top 5 favorite.

Which naughty acts did you play over and over again in your head at work? Which one made you cum the hardest? Which one do you want to try again until you can perfect it?

On the next page, write them down and take turns reading them to each other, one by one.

Top 5 SEX CHALLENGES

HER TOP 5:

1 ....

2 ....

3 ....

4 ....

5 ....

HIS TOP 5:

1 ....

2 ....

3 ....

4 ....

5 ....

THE SEXY TOY
wishlist

Collect all the toys and accessories I've mentioned in this book (plus a few extras) to unlock the most intimate experiences with your partner...

THE BEST VIBRATOR

THE BEST VIBRATOR DURING PLAY

THE REMOTE CONTROL VIBRATOR

SENSUAL MASSAGE OIL

THE BEST LUBE

ROUGH SEX STARTER KIT

TIES FOR THE BED POSTS

LEATHER PADDLE FOR SPANKING

SEXY CANDLES TO SET THE MOOD

PILLOW ASSIST   ANAL TRAINER KIT   HANDCUFFS

SEXY MAID COSTUME   SEXY LOLLIPOPS   WHIPPED CREAM

LIBIDO SUPPORT   COCONUT OIL   SEX DICE

---

want more?

THE BEST SEX TOYS AND ACCESSORIES ARE HERE.

YOUR NEW NAUGHTY CHALLENGE?

To explore the sexual experiences above, weaving them in your normal sex life…that is, if you can consider your sex life "normal" anymore.

Cut out 16 pieces of paper – 8 pieces each. Use each slip of paper to write your Top 5 sex challenges and 3 sex challenges that you'd like to try again.

Fold the papers and put them into a decorative bowl or a fishbowl. As often as you'd like, take turns picking a piece of paper out of the bowl and acting out whatever is on that slip of paper.

important!

Designate at least two solid nights a week to do this. Write it on a calendar and do not skip it.

Prioritize each other. Prioritize your sex life.

DID YOU LOVE THE SEX BUCKET LIST?

Please leave us a review on Amazon.

Help other couples revive their dull sex life!

We're trying to start a sexual revolution here!

sexy notes

sexy notes

Printed in Great Britain
by Amazon